ULTIMATE LEAN MUSCLE MASTERPLAN

a comprehensive guide to building
the ultimate male physique

Adebola Akiyode

Published by PFZ Media

Copyright © 2019 Adebola Akiyode

PREFACE

Building lean muscle is not as complicated as the fitness industry would like you to believe.

Contrary to popular belief, you DO NOT need to spend unreasonable amounts of money buying worthless supplements endorsed by steroid-fuelled bodybuilders, spend countless hours doing ineffective exercises every single day, or obsess over excessively restrictive diets to get your dream physique.

This book explains exactly how you can build muscle effectively with a lean bulk. Maybe you're a beginner and you want to start lifting, or you have been lifting for a while but not seeing the results that you are after. This book concisely explains exactly how to start off right, stay on track and attain the physique of your dreams.

You will learn the correct way to approach the essential aspect of nutrition with regard to building a lean, muscular body. You will also learn an all-in-one training routine that delivers MAXIMUM results for your efforts, helping you to build a big full chest, a wide tapered back, thick powerful legs, and bulging arms, while spending no more than 3 - 6 hours in the gym every week.

NUTRITION

When most gym goers think about the concept of "bulking", they think it means 'eat everything in sight because the more food I consume the more muscle I will grow'. That, unfortunately, is **NOT** how the body operates physiologically. If anything, excessive calories are more easily stored as body fat than as extra muscle tissue. It is therefore important to do things properly to make sure you gain as much muscle as possible while minimizing fat gain.

In this chapter, I will dive into the nutritional aspect of a lean bulk. Subsequent chapters will discuss training techniques, mind-set development and guidelines on how to avoid common mistakes on your quest for lean bulk.

Macronutrients

Many people start following meal plans when they are trying to build muscle and that is not necessarily a wrong approach but I do think it's very important to understand why you do certain things and why it actually works.

Understanding calories and macronutrients are the key to controlling fat loss and muscle gain. The term "macronutrient" describes the major components of someone's diet that are required in relatively large amounts.

The 3 main energy containing macronutrients are:

- Protein,
- Carbohydrates, and
- Fats.

Energy from food macronutrients comes in the form of heat called "Calories". Carbohydrates and proteins contain 4 calories per gram, while fats contain 9 calories per gram. Macronutrients are colloquially referred to as Macros.

Protein

Protein is used by the body to build, repair and maintain muscle tissue. Protein consists of amino acids, which are also referred to as the building blocks of protein.

Protein is essential for the growth and the building of new tissue as well as the repair of broken down tissue, which is exactly what happens to your body when you workout. It is therefore crucial to get the right amount of protein, since your goal is to build muscle.

Some examples of protein sources are lean beef, chicken, fish, turkey, eggs, beans, and tofu, to name a few.

Fats

Fats, technically called 'lipids', are the most energy dense of the 3 macronutrients. They are composed of building blocks called "fatty acids". A fat-free diet can hinder muscle growth in a person who exercises. Consequently, it is very important that you get a sufficient amount of fats each day. Fats can be obtained from different sources, some of these include olive oil, avocados, nuts, chia seeds, butter and cheese.

Carbohydrates

Carbohydrates (colloquially known as carbs) have come to have quite a bad reputation in recent times, especially as 'low-carb' foods have gained popularity. Many people think that carbohydrates are the enemy and that they are the primary cause of body-fat gain. This is incorrect.

Carbohydrates are the preferred fuel source for your body's and brain's energy needs. It is carbohydrate energy that fuels your workouts. If you want to build muscle, you must make sure that you have enough fuel to progress in the gym.

Too many calories of any type can lead to fat gain. With carbohydrates, people consume too many sugary carb-rich foods which also often contain fats. While your body needs carbohydrates for fuel and energy, be mindful that it only needs a limited amount.

A few examples of foods that are rich in carbohydrates are whole grains, pasta, rice, bread, potatoes, yams, and fruits.

Micronutrients and Fibre

Micronutrients are parts of foods that do not provide caloric energy, but still perform a range of physiological duties, and are vital to maintaining optimum health. Micronutrients include vitamins, minerals and organic acids.

Most people do not need to track their micronutrient intake as long as they are eating a sufficient amount of fruits and vegetable on a daily basis.

Fibre is another important component of a healthy person's diet. Fibre helps the digestive process, assists with mineral balance, improves heart health, and improves blood lipids.

Hydration

Many people are not aware of how water affects their performance. Even being slightly dehydrated can cause poor performance and is, sadly, often overlooked. I recommend drinking between 3 and 4 litres of water every day.

Why track Macros instead of Calories?

Calories are not all the same. A calorie is a unit of measurement that represents the amount of energy your body gains upon consumption. You must, however, consider the source of these calories. Two foods may have similar calorie content but completely different macronutrient and micronutrient breakdowns. For example, 300 calories of doughnuts are likely to have a different effect on your mental and physical state than 300 calories of apples. Therefore, I would highly recommend that you track your macronutrients and not just your calories.

How to calculate your daily Macros

There are many free tools on the internet and mobile app stores that can help you calculate your personal Macros. In using any of these tools, make sure that they contain a TDEE Calculator. TDEE is an acronym for "Total Daily Energy Expenditure" and it refers to the amount of calories you burn each day. Therefore, if your TDEE matches the amount of calories you consume in a day, your body mass will remain the same. TDEE is also known as 'maintenance calories' because it is the amount of calories you need to maintain your current body mass. If you consume more calories than your TDEE, you are likely to gain weight and if you consume less calories than your TDEE, you will lose weight over time.

In order to do a lean bulk, you have to consume more calories than you burn. This is called being in a caloric surplus. The reverse is eating in a caloric deficit, which as explained above, is when you eat less calories than you burn - leading to a loss of body fat (also called 'cutting').

For the purposes that this book is written to address, we will concentrate on eating in a caloric surplus to build muscle. The reason we refer to 'lean bulk' is because you will only be in a very **slight** caloric surplus as opposed to eating a lot more food than your body can burn. This minimizes fat gain and makes sure you mainly gain muscle.

The concept basically is that when you are eating at maintenance, you will stay the same regardless of your workout. When you eat a little more, your body will use that extra food energy to build extra muscle. If you overindulge in food, your body will start to accumulate fat. Similarly, if you eat much less food than the energy you use in a day, your body will not be able to sustain its current shape and it will therefore start to burn fat from your body's reserves as energy.

It is generally better to concentrate on building a lean bulk until you have attained a sufficient amount of muscle. When you have a built a decent amount of muscle, you can start cutting to get lean by entering a caloric deficit.

You can start calculating your daily Macros by learning your TDEE and adding 200 calories (the surplus) to that number. My TDEE at a weight of 90 kilograms, for example, is 2,700 calories. By adding 200 calories, to create a caloric surplus, my TDEE for a lean bulk comes to a total of 2,900 calories.

I enter 2,900 calories into my Macro calculator as my daily caloric target and click on 'calculate' to see a breakdown of the recommended daily quantity of Macros that is ideal for my goal. This calculation will usually recommend that I consume 166 grams of protein, 64 grams of fat, and 414 grams of carbohydrates per day.

Take note that these numbers will vary from person to person because every body is different and every body needs a different amount of calories per day. Also take notice that the numbers generated by any calculator are only a rough estimate because macro calculators cannot take some other influential factors into account.

Macro calculators are, however, a very good tool with which to start; even though you may need a human coach to consider your special needs and guide you through the lean bulk journey.

Tracking your food intake

Now you have the numbers, what is next?

Every food that you eat contains a certain number of calories and macronutrients (proteins, carbohydrates and fats). The goal is to hit the macronutrient targets set by your calculations every single day. In order to do this effectively, you should track your food intake by entering every food you eat into your Macro calculator. You do not have to keep doing this indefinitely if you do not want to, but you surely have to do it at the beginning of your lean bulk journey to get an understanding of the foods you eat regularly and their macronutrient profiles.

A good macronutrient calculator is the 'myfitnesspal' app, which is free to download on all major mobile app stores.

Every food contains a different amount of protein, fats and carbs. It is therefore not possible to eat some foods in large amounts, as it will lead to the over-consumption of one macronutrient over the others.

It is typically very difficult to hit your set Macros every single day, and this is fine. Try to be within a 5 to 10-gram ratio of your targets and you will still see your desired results. For example, if your target for protein is 170 grams a day, it is fine for you to consume 180 grams of protein in a day. It is also fine to consume 160 grams in one day.

When you purchase food at a grocery store, most will have a label that contains information on the food's macronutrient contents. Before you eat a food, weigh it out and enter the food into your Macro calculator. I recommend weighing and entering into the calculator before you actually eat the food, so that you can see what the effect will be on the numbers, before consumption.

You might make some mistakes in the beginning because you do not have sufficient knowledge about the different macronutrients of food sources and, therefore, you may eat too much of one by accident. Making mistakes is part of the process of learning.

As hinted above, you can manually enter food names into the calculator and search for macronutrient information within most calculators, or you can scan the barcode on the food packet. You should always double-check with the label of the food to see if the macronutrients are equal to the information that the Macro calculator generates. As users can manually enter information into Macro calculators, sometimes errors are made, hence the emphasis on double checking.

Many people decide to follow a meal plan, eating the same foods in the same quantities every single day. This is a good way to track your daily macronutrients since it involves less thinking and juggling of numbers, as you only have to calculate your Macros once.

You can eat any food you want as long as you hit your macronutrients of the day. Most active individuals, however, stand to get the most out of their training and lifestyle by consuming nutrient-dense, minimally processed foods. This includes foods like whole grains, vegetables, fruits, lean meats, nuts, eggs, certain dairy products and not too much processed foods. I typically recommend a diet of around 80-90% whole unprocessed foods and 10-20% processed foods. This will help you to accommodate any cravings you may have and ensure that you can keep the right balance and live your best life while getting in shape. The fitness journey is supposed to be fun and should not take over your life. Instead, it should enhance your life.

It is absolutely possible to maintain a correct balance, enjoy your life to the fullest and get in great shape at the same time.

These are the nutritional basics on how to start a lean bulk. In the next chapter, I will explain everything you need to know in order to build a build muscle in the gym.

TRAINING

Gym goers usually experience lack of knowledge, confusion, and misinformation from following bodybuilding magazines or listening to the 'biggest guy in the gym' without actually thinking twice. This could give you some results, depending on whether the advice given is correct, but very often, it is not.

Sometimes, even wrong advice on training can show results at the start because the beginner is excited to train and his body will change to adapt to new stimuli. He will, however, find that progress stalls really quickly and consequently will have a hard time taking his physique to the next level of fitness.

Getting results in the gym is not always about working hard. It is also about working smart.

The typical workout routine for most gym goers looks like this:

Monday	-	**Chest and Triceps**
Tuesday	-	**Back and Biceps**
Wednesday	-	**Rest**
Thursday	-	**Legs**
Friday	-	**Shoulders**
Saturday	-	**Rest**
Sunday	-	**Rest**

Or like this:

Monday	-	**Chest**
Tuesday	-	**Back**
Wednesday	-	**Legs**
Thursday	-	**Shoulders**
Friday	-	**Arms**
Saturday	-	**Rest**
Sunday	-	**Rest**

For natural lifters in general, and especially for beginners, this is not an effective way to train. It usually involves very high volume training, one body part per week, training to failure, a lot of supersets and drop sets, and a lot of isolation exercises.

As alluded to above, the origin of these routines is usually from bodybuilding publications or as advertised by popular professional bodybuilders. First of all, it is important to note that these bodybuilders are on a completely different level of training than the average gym user and it does not make sense to train using their techniques and plans. Secondly, many bodybuilders use anabolic steroids and this makes them able to train in a completely different way than those who train naturally.

The more effective method, suitable for beginners, includes less volume per workout and a higher frequency of training per week.

Which workout should you do?

I have created a 3-day routine for you that I recommend beginners to follow, as well as those who have not had great results in the gym despite their dedication. You might not feel like you are a beginner, but if you have been training the wrong way for sometime, I would recommend that you give this routine a try.

Good news! You do **not** have to hit the gym every single day. Many people that start lifting think that more is better but that is not the case. Less is often more. Your body needs rest and since this routine contains a lot of big lifts, it is very tasking on your central nervous system, and thus too intense to do every day.

Another reason that this workout plan is better for beginners is that because the lean bulk journey brings a radically different shift to your lifestyle, it will inevitably require a lot of effort to form into a routine and, therefore may lead to skipped sessions or quitting. This plan is simple enough to ensure that it is not too rigorous for beginners while being extremely effective.

I recommend that you start this routine 3 times a week and once you can keep it up for a while, you should move up to the 4-day and 5-day workout plans also available in this series.

In following the 3-day routine, you should spread the sessions throughout the week with at least one day of rest between each session. You will be training your whole body in each workout and therefore will need at least 1 day to recover properly for the next session.

In the beginning, all the major muscle groups will be targeted in each workout. You will not split them throughout the week. By doing big compound lifts, you will get the most value out of your workout and you will get as strong as you possibly can in a relatively short period of time. The progression is amazing on this routine and it is therefore the best for beginners.

If you have been following a similar routine to one of the two shown at the beginning of this chapter, and you give this full body routine a try, you will see your progress skyrocket in the gym.

The Set-up of the Routine

I would usually recommend that you adopt the routine by training on Mondays, Wednesdays and Fridays with the full weekend to rest. You can, however, decide to structure the days differently as long as you have 1 day of rest in between each session (e.g. Training on Tuesdays, Thursdays and Saturdays).

You will switch between A and B workouts, and so workouts will be on different days each week.

Warming-Up

Before you start your workout, it is very important to properly warm-up first. A good warm-up will take about 10-15 minutes and will make sure that your whole body is in a proper state to lift heavy weights. It will also help you to avoid injuries and therefore should not be skipped. I recommend using the following warmup routine:

Rolling arm forward:	**10 times**
Rolling arm backwards:	**10 times**
Scapular Push ups:	**20 times**
Scapular Pull Ups:	**10 times**
Leg swing to side:	**10 times each leg**
Leg swing to front:	**10 times each leg**
Cable side external rotation:	**10 times / 2 sets**
Cable up external rotation:	**10 times / 2 sets**

The Workouts

The difference between A and B workouts is that A has a main focus of building strength, while B is focused towards hypertrophy, also known as muscle growth. A combination of both workouts will inevitably ensure that you gain both strength and mass a result of your exercise. The best way to implement workouts A and B is as follows:

Monday	**(Day 1)**	**Workout A**
Tuesday		
Wednesday	**(Day 2)**	**Workout B**
Thursday		
Friday	**(Day 3)**	**Workout A**
Saturday		
Sunday		
Monday	**(Day 4)**	**Workout B**

Workout A

This is a strength workout and will require that you do relatively low repetitions (or "reps") to focus on getting as strong as you can. The reps will still be high enough to also aid your muscle building goals. The rest time in between sets is higher than that required of Workout B.

I recommend doing 1-2 quick warm-up sets before you get into your actual weight on each body part. You may need more warm-up sets depending on how heavy you can go.

You can find specific visual guidance on all individual exercises in the form of tutorial videos on YouTube or other online resources.

Workout A is as follows:

Exercise	Reps	Sets	Rest (minutes)
Squat	3 – 5	4	2
Deadlift	3 – 5	2	2
Bench Press	3 – 5	4	2
Weighted Pullups	3 – 5	4	2
Overhead Press	3 – 5	3	2
Barbell Curl	6 – 8	3	1
Skull Crusher	6 – 8	3	1
Rope Crunch	10-12	5	1

Workout B

This is a hypertrophy workout and this will require relatively higher reps. You will also be doing more volume in total in this workout. The rest time in between sets is lower than that on Workout A.

Make sure you put your timer on after you complete a set so that you do not rest for too long or too little. It is important to stick to the program setup.

Workout B is as follows:

Exercise	Reps	Sets	Rest (minutes)
Squat	8 – 10	4	1.5
Stiff Legged Deadlift	8 – 10	4	1.5
Incline Dumbbell Press	8 – 10	4	1.5
Bent Over Row	8 – 10	4	1.5
Dumbbell Seated Overhead Press	8 – 10	2	1
Standing Lateral Raises	10 – 12	2	1
Tricep Pushdown	10 – 12	3	1
Incline Hammer Curls	10 – 12	3	1
Weighted Knee Raises	12 – 15	5	1

You will notice that, on the routines, there is a focus on isolation lifts compared to other publicized routines and this has to do with the fact that the routine in this book was created with the intention of building and developing an aesthetic physique. Strength is one of the goals, but the main target is to transform the way that you look.

Progressive overload

Progressive overload is the key to muscle growth. It means the gradual increase of stress placed on the body during exercise. It is a very simple concept to understand and means that you must continually place more stress on your body to give it a reason to grow.

The goal on your lifts is to start with a set weight in a lower repetition (or 'rep') range and keep the weight the same while doing more reps until the end of the rep range is reached. From there, you will add weight and then go back to the lower end of the rep range and repeat.

Keep in mind that everyone progresses at a different rate due to many factors. As long as you are adding some weight or some reps to the exercise, you are doing well and you will make gains.

Tracking your workouts

Many beginners go to the gym and train hard but do not track their workouts. They do different weights and reps each time and focus on chasing "the pump". Even though the pump feels nice, just like muscle soreness the day after a workout, these are not indicators of muscle growth. Real progression is made by training smart.

Track your workouts in order to progressively overload. Apps like 'rep-count' are a good way to keep track of your workout. These give you a game plan and make it easy to know exactly what you need to do when you get into the gym. Tracking your workouts optimizes your time and effort while training.

De-loading

De-loading is 'taking one step back in order to take two steps forward'. People often de-load or take weeks off when they reach a persistent state of fatigue. If you have reached this point, you are already too late. You may find yourself overreaching, not making progress, or even getting weaker and potentially getting injured.

De-loading is done to prevent overreaching, weakness and injuries from happening and to ensure that you make steady progress. It is very important and must not be skipped.

After 6-10 weeks of following this program, you should include a de-load week. A de-load week every 6-8 weeks of training is recommended for older people or experienced lifters, while beginners should take a de-load week after every 8-10 weeks of training.

During a de-load week, you will simply do only 60% of the amount of sets of the regular workout. You should also use 60% of the weights required for each exercise. The rest time and the amount of rest should stay the same.

This chapter covers everything you need to know to start training the right way if you are a beginner or if you have previously not been training properly.

Once you have been training using this routine for a long period of time, you should ideally switch to one of the 4-day or 5-day workout plans also available in this series.

MIND-SET DEVELOPMENT

So far in this book, I have given you all the essential knowledge needed to build an aesthetically pleasing body. You should now know what and how to eat, as well as how to train effectively. All you need to do is to follow the simple steps provided every single day.

Despite the fact that this sounds so simple, it is in fact not easy. In fact, this is the main reason why most people on planet earth are not in great shape. Even though all the steps are super simple to break down, an essential ingredient for the attainment of ANY goal is having the proper state of mind.

Getting in shape requires a lot of discipline and this chapter will guide you through this aspect of your journey.

When it comes to getting in shape, it is the making of many decisions on a daily basis that will affect your progress and, ultimately your results.

In the morning, will you really wake up earlier to hit the gym before going to your workplace? Or do you hear that alarm, feel tired and decide to keep sleeping?

If someone offers you that doughnut during lunch and everybody takes one, will you refuse it because you are trying to get in shape?

When your friends want to go to the movies at night but you have a workout planned, will you skip the gym to join them? Or will you complete your workout session instead?

There is nothing wrong with eating doughnuts or hanging out with your friends, but you do have to set priorities if you want to be successful on your journey to an aesthetically pleasing body.

You have to make rules for yourself so that you do not constantly go off track. If you cannot successfully take care of your own body, your chances of success in any other aspect of your life become quite slim.

If you constantly slack, you give up, you disappoint yourself and are not able to keep to the rules you have set for your own self, how are you possibly going to be a winner?

Getting in shape and working on your physical health is the best possible investment you can make in yourself for the rest of your life. The beginning of this journey is the toughest part, and this is where most people quit. If you can push through the beginning, however, the journey becomes a lot easier.

You can develop the correct mind-set to attain your desired results by following these steps:

Step 1

Take a photograph of yourself in your current shape. It is important that you have a basis to compare your new self with your old self. This is a key driver of progress and is very likely to motivate you. I recommend taking progress photographs or videos once a week.

It is unlikely that you will see massive visual changes every week, but after many weeks and months, you definitely will. You might not even realise how much you have changed until you compare these photographs and/or videos with each other.

Step 2

Take regular measurements of your body and start to weigh your-self every morning. Measurements can be taken every month, but weighing should be done every morning. You should take the average of 7 days' weight to give yourself a weekly number for your body's weight. This way, you can track your progress in weight loss or weight gain as in our case.

Step 3

Write down your specific goals. This may sound cliché, but re-search in neuroscience proves that writing down goals makes it significantly more likely that they will be achieved. Your goals must be specific and must have a deadline (e.g. within the next 90 days, I want to drop 6 kilograms of weight).

Step 4

Write down a specific plan. These are the daily actions that you will have to execute in order to reach your goal (e.g. I will go to the gym and lift weights 3 times a week; I will do cardiovascular exercises for 30 minutes after each workout and High Intensity Interval Training on one of my rest days; I will eat X amount of calories every day; I will only drink alcohol once a week).

You are responsible for your accountability in attaining these goals. If you find it extremely difficult to stay accountable, I recommend hiring a coach physically or on the internet.

Step 5

Plan out your week, making sure that you have set days on which you will workout at the gym, and preferably at the same time each week to form a habit. If you have an irregular schedule, make sure to plan your day the night before.

You have to see training and eating your meals as a priority. You must complete these tasks before you declare that you have any free time.

Meal-prepping is an effective way to ensure that you manage your time easily.

If you slip on your journey, do not dismay. Simply accept that you did not attain your goal for that day and move on to the next day neither trying to make your diet worse by binge eating nor better by starving.

Motivation vs Discipline

Motivation comes and goes and will not always be there to help you stay on track. On some days, you just will not feel like sticking to the script and it is important to recognise this. Successful people understand that discipline is what matters in order to attain big goals. It is not something that you are born with, it is self learned behaviour.

Discipline is essential quality necessary to maintain the correct mindset for achieving your fitness goals.

Comparing yourself to others

In today's world, it is easier to compare oneself with others than it has ever been in history. With easy access to social media platforms, it is common for people starting a fitness journey to be overwhelmed by all the amazing physiques that they may want to look like. You, however, must remember that someone else's Chapter 10 will be completely different to your Chapter 1.

Every body starts somewhere, and since you only see the results - not the full span - of other people's journeys, it is not fair or reasonable to compare yourself with others. Instead, you should compare yourself with your previous self.

It is You vs You.

Look back at your previous photographs, see your progress and take pride in it.

How to live with judgment

Whenever you decide to do something for yourself, it inevitably attracts the judgment of other people. When I started my fitness journey, I was slightly chubby, insecure and downright ashamed of my physical appearance. As I took fitness more seriously, I was scorned and teased by many of my peers, making my journey lonelier and consequently, more difficult. I was called names in jest such as 'Mr Macho', 'Incredible Hulk' and even 'Freak'.

Judgment really says more about the person expressing it than it does about you. It is a horrible thing to judge people especially when they are visibly trying to improve themselves as in this case. It is, however, sadly unavoidable in human societies.

Try to surround yourself with positive people. Where this is not absolutely possible, you should realise that you are in this journey alone, it is your life and your decision to improve it, therefore, you must ignore the judgment of other people.

Patience

Patience is another key when it comes to developing the right mind-set for your fitness journey. You must understand that fitness is a marathon and not a sprint. It is not about reaching some short term goal, but about creating a lifestyle to be followed forever.

Many people that get into fitness only picture the end goal or dream result. They obsess about the end physique and what they want to look like and forget to actually enjoy the process of fitness. Life is all about the journey. It is about all your ups and downs on your way to achieving your dreams, and the same thing goes for fitness.

You should concentrate on enjoying every step and taking in all the compliments you receive on the way.

Patience is very essential as it is going to take a long time to achieve your goals. No matter how much you try, you cannot work harder in order to outwork the need for patience. With patience, you will develop a healthy mind-set to ensure that you enjoy every step of your fitness journey.

Accepting fat gain

Building muscle is very different from losing weight. It is a relatively slow process and you are unlikely to see big visual changes in a short period of time. With fat loss, you may see rapid welcome changes in a matter of weeks and more progress on a weekly basis, but in building muscle, you can sometimes begin to look worse while you work towards your goal.

This is because your body will hold a little more fat and you will likely retain water weight while you go through your caloric surplus. You may therefore not look better over the initial months of your lean bulk compared to when you're losing fat, but you must mentally remind yourself that this is a normal phase in the grand scheme of investing in yourself. You must assure yourself that when it is time for you to shred fat by cutting, you will look the best that you have ever done.

Balance

I cannot overemphasize the importance of maintaining a healthy balance in your fitness journey. A lack of balance is a major factor behind why many people do not attain positive results. People are always looking for the next best "secret" that will get them in shape quickly.

Some programs, especially weight loss programs, can give you rapid results but are not sustainable in the long run. Starvation diets and other similar trends, for example, are not balanced and will ensure that any gains experienced are lost within a short amount of time.

You must allow yourself to still be able to go out with loved ones, party and eat nice foods. Doing these will create a sustainable life-style pattern and should ensure that you have more fun on your fitness journey.

Balance refers to living a great life while getting in shape.

All of the above may sound boring, serious and even arduous. Welcome to reality! The inability to keep up with these is why most people are not in shape. Fitness takes a lot of time, effort, blood, sweat and tears, but it is all worth it at the end of the day because you will achieve something that most people do not have.

If you want to accomplish something that most people do not have, you must be willing to do things that most people are not willing to do. Stop procrastinating, start taking action, realise that your life is in your hands, and it is what you make it.

Let's stop being victims and start being winners.

DO NOT BACK TRACK!

In this chapter, I will discuss 7 of the biggest mistakes made in trying to build lean mass. Reading this chapter should ensure that you are able to determine when you are doing anything detrimental to your fitness journey and will let you know how to fix any mistakes. The 7 major mistakes that fitness enthusiasts make, in my experience, are as follows:

Over-eating

Eating whatever you like whenever you like is a common mistake. As mentioned in the chapter on nutrition above, many people wrongly believe that whatever they eat goes straight into their muscles, and the more they eat, the better. This is not correct!

Over-eating to put on weight is colloquially called a 'dirty bulk'. The issue with a dirty bulk or unstructured bulk is that although you may attain an impressive size and gain strength in the gym, it is all an illusion because a lot of the weight you put on is as a result of fat mass and water retention.

You can avoid over-eating by tracking your Macros and staying disciplined in doing so.

Under-eating

Conversely, not eating enough while trying to lean bulk will hamper your journey towards attaining an aesthetically pleasing lean bulk. You are more likely to under-eat if you do not closely monitor your calorie intake. You can therefore ensure that you are always on the right track by calculating and tracking your Macros as explained in the chapter on nutrition.

Not bulking for long enough

This is a common mistake that people make because when you are very lean, especially coming out of a cutting phase, you will gain some fat in the process and your muscle definition may not be as sharp as it once was. This 'fatty' appearance does not have much to do with the actual body fat you have put on, but the glycogen and the water that your body is holding.

If you experience this, you must not get impatient or panic and cut your bulking phase prematurely. You must, instead, trust the process and stick with it to ensure that you put on the right amount of muscle mass in order to attain the physique of your dreams. Rest assured that, with discipline, you will easily do away with any unnecessary fat deposits on your body during your cutting phase.

Consuming too much protein

When you read fitness magazines or look at a bodybuilder's meal plan, there will usually be a lot of protein in it. The reason for this is that these bodybuilders use steroids to enhance their muscle growth and so they need an unusual amount of protein.

As a natural bodybuilder, you cannot absorb as much protein as a bodybuilder on steroids, so it does not make sense to follow the same regimen. The reality is that once your protein intake is high enough, your body will not use any excess protein effectively. Some people think that the body will automatically excrete the excess protein, but this is not the case. Your body will attempt to convert it into energy and will do so inefficiently, which will have detrimental effects on your physique.

Not sticking to a goal

This is a very common mistake that I have fallen victim to many times in the past.

You want to gain muscle but whilst you are doing this, a few months in, you start to feel that you are not as muscular and aesthetic anymore. You do not see your veins popping out and your abdominal muscles only show in very low resolution, so you feel the need to start cutting again prematurely. After cutting for a while, you miss your bulk and start to chase the dream of bigger muscles again. This cycle goes on and on and your mind will continue to play these games with you.

The reality is that, being human, you are unlikely to be happy with wherever you are and the grass is always greener on the other side.

Set a goal, completely focus on it, enjoy the process and achieve your target!

Over-training

I have also been guilty of this mistake many times and it is the one mistake I am most likely to repeat.

At the end of every workout session, I would usually feel excess energy and attempt to push myself to failure without sticking to my plan. This has the detrimental effect of putting unnecessary stress on the body and taking away some benefit from your future sessions.

When you practice progressive overload, you should do so strategically and within a defined structure.

It is very important to keep training smart and not just hard.

Eating a lot of junk food

I understand that after you have completed a cutting phase where you intensely restricted yourself in terms of calories consumed, you may want to eat every single thing in sight. It is fine to let yourself go for a day or two but you must remain disciplined and call yourself to reality as quickly as possible.

Some people see the bulking phase as an opportunity to eat large amounts of junk food because they have a lot of calories to fill up. A popular saying is "a calorie is a calorie regardless of where you get it". This is not correct!

It definitely does matter where you get your calories from. If you eat junk food predominantly, you will not feel good mentally. This means that your workouts will not go as well as they possibly could. It also means that you will not find your fitness journey as enjoyable as you possibly can.

You should ensure that your diet is balanced and contains fibre, water, vitamins and minerals. The ultimate goal is not just to build muscle but to be healthy, to look good and to feel good in the process.

GOOD LUCK!!!

www.ingramcontent.com/pod-product-compliance
Lightning Source LLC
Chambersburg PA
CBHW051428250726
48655CB00003B/1295